Bon Voyage: Traveling with Essent [...]
project. Traveling to 24 countries a [...]
U.S. over the years has led me to c [...]
best protect me from germs and foreign invaders my body is not
accustomed to handling.

Through extensive research and volunteer testers like my
daughter, many Young Living members, and myself, I conclude
that Young Living™ Essential Oils really work! They are easy to
transport, easy to use and very versatile. You may find you do
best with a different selection of oils than what works for me.
That's okay; use what works for you. I am very thankful that we
have an abundance of quality oils from which to choose. In the
back of this booklet there is a page for you to keep notes and
record specific recipes and combinations you put together for
your personal travel needs.

This booklet will provide ideas, recommendations, and
suggestions to help you travel with your essential oils with ease.
However as you will notice upon reading, this work is considered
third-party noncompliant material. Please follow the Young Living
guidelines in accordance with their policies and procedures about
posting and sharing noncompliant material.

With a little planning and preparation you will be able to enjoy
your travels, see sites and wonders in person, and create lasting
memories for you and your family without the worry of getting
sick on your adventures.

Happy, healthy travels to you,

Debra

Debra Raybern

Bon Voyage

Getting ready to go somewhere special? Perhaps you are setting off for the sunny beaches of the Caribbean, the snowy mountains of Colorado, the backwoods of Tennessee, a week-long cruise, a road trip across your state or a bus ride with fellow conventioneers. You've planned your trip, and now it's time to pack your bags.

What will you take with you? Will you bring only a carry-on bag or opt for checked baggage? Whether driving in a car or bus, flying, going by train, or sailing in a boat, you're sure to want a stash of essential oils and other items within easy reach to defend your body against foreign invaders, support your digestive system when food choices aren't ideal, and to keep your spirits and energy high amid all the fun.

Traveling with essential oils is a great way to provide protection from the discomforts you might encounter – bad food or water, upset stomach, diarrhea, vomiting, headaches, ear pain from altitude variations, pesky insects, parasites, viruses and bacteria, cuts, scrapes, boo-boos, fatigue, etc. If you are prepared with items on-hand and ready to use while traveling, camping, vacationing or even heading into the mission field, you'll be ready to tackle all scenarios and emergencies.

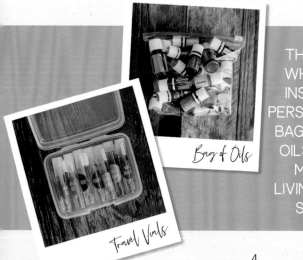

Bag of Oils

Travel Vials

THERE HAVE BEEN TIMES WHEN MY LUGGAGE WAS INSPECTED AND THE TSA PERSONNEL, UPON SEEING MY BAGGIE FULL OF ESSENTIAL OILS, REMARKED, "OH, YOU MUST BE WITH YOUNG LIVING," TO WHICH I ALWAYS SMILE AND SAY, "YES".

TSA Regulations

When traveling by plane, the Transportation Security Administration (TSA) allows one quart-sized bag of liquids, aerosols, gels, creams and pastes in your carry-on bag and through security checkpoints. These are limited to travel-sized containers that are 3.4 ounces (100 mL) or less per item. The TSA categorizes essential oils as liquids. As such, if you want to carry them with you on the plane, they must fit in a single quart-sized bag along with any other liquids you are carrying on with you.

A traditional quart-sized baggie will hold about 18-15 mL bottles of oil. I suggest carrying on only those oils that you need during your flight. Additional essential oils and other liquids travel safely in checked baggage. If you are not checking bags, consider dividing the oils you take with you amongst the other family members or filling several 2 mL sample vials with the oils you will need. However if, like me, you often travel alone, checking a bag with your essential oils may be the best option.

Packing Tips

PLAN AHEAD

There are many essential oils you may wish to take on your trip. Included in this booklet are the ones that my family and I have relied on for years to keep us healthy during our travels. My daughter and I have traveled to 24 countries across North, Central and South America and Europe with NO occurrence of illness. The better prepared you are, the better your chances of avoiding anything that could spoil your vacation. If you are aware of specific circumstances at your destination that could involve risk, be sure to do some research ahead of time and select oils that will help you stay healthy while visiting. Many oils will serve multiple purposes; learn the versatility of the oils and avoid over-packing.

Preparation for traveling should also include ramping up your immune system support a week or two prior to departure and keeping up with a good "protection" program as you travel. As they say, "an ounce of prevention is worth a pound of cure."

I prefer to travel with 5 mL bottles of oils. Some go in my carry-on bag in an approved quart-sized baggie, while others are packed in my checked luggage. Sample vials containing about 10 drops of oils that I use less frequently help to conserve space. The longer the trip, the more oils and supplements I carry. On longer trips and those outside the U.S., I'm certain to bring precautionary items like ParaFree™, Ocotea and DiGize™, whereas a two- or three-day conference within the U.S. warrants fewer necessities. Spend a little time planning what you will need for the length of your trip and destination, and pack your oils and supplements accordingly.

PROTECT YOUR OILS

When packing essential oils in checked baggage, protect them by storing in a padded oil carrier. 5 mL bottles are the most convenient, and larger roll-ons will rest nicely on top. Be sure the caps are securely tightened as they may shift and be upside-down at some point. To prevent bottles from leaking, when they have been previously opened, whether carrying-on or checking, you can place a small piece of plastic wrap over the orifice before securing the cap.

DON'T FORGET THE SUPPLEMENTS

Be sure to bring enough of the supplements on which your family relies. If you are preparing for a relatively short trip, you may be able to pack them in a pill case. Another option is to pack and label your supplements in 2" x 3" resealable bags commonly used for hobbies and crafts. Properly labeled, these can travel in carry-on or checked bags and there is nothing to bring back home. NingXia Red® packets and NingXia Nitro® can be placed in a large zipper bag, or better yet, in a vacuum seal bag. Be sure to bring along a TSA-approved pair of scissors to open vacuum-sealed bags.

WATER, WATER EVERYWHERE AND NOT A DROP TO DRINK!

Especially when traveling abroad, it is advisable to find a filtered water bottle that you can easily carry with you. A quick search online will reveal many choices. This item will take up very little room and will be worth its weight in gold. Remember to empty the bottle and leave the lid off prior to going through the TSA checkpoint, so that it is visibly seen as empty. If available, name brand bottled water is generally safe to drink as well.

Let's Start Packing!

CARRY-ON NECESSITIES

The following is a list of don't-leave-home-without items that you will want to pack in your carry on bag to have handy while in transit. Refer to the "Symptom Guide" (p. 14) for specific usage information.

- **AromaEase™** – prevents and eases motion sickness
- **KidScents® SniffleEase™** – relieves motion sickness in young children; may also help ease symptoms of jet lag
- **Ledum** – relieves motion sickness in adults and children, keeps the lymphatic system functioning, relieves ear pain associated with pressure changes or infection
- **Melrose™** – relieves ear pain from pressure or altitude changes
- **NingXia Red® & Inner Defense™** – combat negative effects of radiation exposure from airport security scans
- **Peppermint or Ginger Vitality™** – prevent and ease motion sickness
- **Sensation™ or Genesis™ Hand & Body Lotion** – keep skin hydrated
- **Slique™ Gum** – chew inflight to relieve ear pressure resulting from altitude changes
- **Stress Away™, Peace & Calming®, or Tranquil™ Roll-On** – use to relieve stress, anxiety, and/or fear of flying in adults or children

12 JUN 2011
HEATHROW (94)

- **Thieves® Spray or Thieves® Wipes** – use to disinfect tray table, armrests, headrests, knobs, handles, buttons, etc.
- **Thieves® Hand Purifier** – use frequently to combat germs.

BE SENSITIVE TO OTHER PASSENGERS

Other travelers do not always appreciate strong smells from essential oils onboard a plane, train, bus, or other crowded vehicle. Applying the oils you want BEFORE boarding allows that first noticeable smell to dissipate so other passengers will not complain.

ESSENTIAL OILS

Below is a list of essential oils that will address many needs during travel. Refer to the "Symptom Guide" (p. 14) for specific usage information and to decide which oils you will need for your particular excursion.

- **AnimalScents™ RepelAroma™** – can be added to YL Insect Repellent for added protection against insects
- **AromaEase™** – prevents and eases motion sickness
- **Cedarwood** – promotes brain function and relieves jet lag; prevents and eases altitude sickness
- **Deep Relief™ Roll-On** – soothes sore muscles, aches, pains, and joint stiffness; apply to injuries for relief of pain and to speed healing
- **DiGize™/DiGize™ Vitality™** – alleviate all types of digestive discomfort, including overeating, heartburn, indigestion, bloating, food poisoning, diarrhea, gas, dry heaves, or constipation; may also use to disinfect cuts and scrapes
- **EndoFlex™ Vitality™** – relieves jet lag; gives you a burst of energy.
- **Eucalyptus Blue** – use for respiratory comfort.
- **Frankincense/Frankincense Vitality™** – combine with Idaho Balsam Fir and Lemon Vitality™ for bladder/kidney support; calms nerves; wear as perfume; use to anoint others when praying.
- **Ginger Vitality™** – prevents and eases motion sickness.
- **Helichrysum** – use to quickly stop bleeding.
- **Idaho Balsam Fir** – combine with Frankincense Vitality™ and Lemon Vitality™ for bladder/kidney support.

- **JuvaFlex®/JuvaFlex® Vitality™** – can bring relief from digestive complaints resulting from overindulgence of food or alcohol.
- **Lavender** – apply to insect bites to relieve pain and promote healing; relieves ear pain from infection or swimmer's ear; calming and relaxing to both parents and children; helps promote a restful night's sleep; may relieve headaches; eases jet lag; apply to injuries for relief of pain and to speed healing.
- **Ledum** – relieves motion sickness, keeps the lymphatic system functioning properly, relieves ear pain associated with pressure changes or infection.
- **Lemon/Lemon Vitality™** – combine with Frankincense Vitality™ and Idaho Balsam Fir for bladder/kidney support; add to drinking water to alkalize and purify; may guard against malaria and other parasites.
- **Melrose™** – apply to insect bites, cuts, and scrapes to relieve pain and promote healing; relieves ear pain from altitude changes, infection or swimmer's ear; prevents/treats athlete's foot from using communal showers.
- **Mountain Savory** – protects against germs or unwanted pathogens; apply to cuts and scrapes to speed healing and prevent infection, specifically bacterial.
- **Ocotea** – guards against parasites; promotes blood sugar balance; eases digestive concerns. May be used by adults and children.
- **Palo Santo** – use to relieve a dry, scratchy throat.
- **PanAway®** – soothes sore muscles, aches and pains. Apply to injuries for relief of pain and to speed healing.
- **Peace & Calming®** – relieves anxiety in adults and children.
- **Peppermint/Peppermint Vitality™** – energizes, relieves exhaustion, and eases jet lag; alleviates all types of digestive discomfort, including motion sickness, overeating, heartburn, indigestion, bloating, etc.; can be used to relieve a fever in adults and children; prevents and eases altitude sickness.
- **Purification®** – apply to insect bites to relieve pain and promote healing.
- **R.C.™ or Raven™** – eases breathing difficulties and coughing related to high altitude or at the onset of

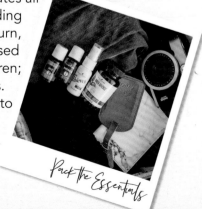

Pack the Essentials

respiratory infection; acts as an expectorant when applied to the chest; promotes improved oxygen uptake and assists the body to expel mucus when inhaled; can be used to disinfect cuts or wounds.
- **Roman Chamomile** – apply to insect bites to relieve pain and promote healing.
- **Stress Away™** – relieves stress and anxiety.
- **Thieves®/Thieves® Vitality™** – supports health of the immune system, combats germs and other pathogens, can be used to draw out glass or splinters imbedded in the skin.
- **Tranquil™ Roll-On** – relieves stress and anxiety.
- **Tsuga** – use to quickly stop bleeding.
- **Valor®** – can be either invigorating or calming; eases fear and anxiety.
- **White Angelica™** – relieves stress, anxiety, and over-stimulation.

SUPPLEMENTS

In addition to your regular supplements, carry the following supplements to combat common issues and remain healthy while traveling. Refer to the "Symptom Guide" (p. 14) for specific usage information.
- **ComforTone® Capsules** – relieve travelers' constipation.
- **Inner Defense™** – protects against the flu, colds, other communicable illness, and free-radical damage.
- **NingXia Nitro®** – restores energy and promotes mental alertness.
- **NingXia Red®** – supports healthy immune system function, alleviates allergic reactions to insect stings, eases travel fatigue, combats a sudden onset of illness, and protects against negative radiation exposure from flying.
- **ParaFree™** – prevents and eliminates parasites.
- **Sleep Essence™** – promotes restful sleep.

PERSONAL CARE PRODUCTS AND OTHER ITEMS
- **Bon Voyage Travel Pack** – a handy pack that contains travel-sized bottles of: Thieves® AromaBright Toothpaste, Thieves® Waterless Hand Purifier, Thieves® Dental Floss, Thieves® Fresh Essence Plus Mouthwash, Young Living Toothbrush, Lavender

Shampoo, Lavender Conditioner, Cinnamint™ Lip Balm, Morning Start™ Bath & Shower Gel, Genesis™ Hand & Body Lotion, ART® Light Moisturizer.

- **Clear Vegetable Capsules** – use for taking oils internally.
- **Insect Repellent**
- **LavaDerm™ After-Sun Spray** – relieves pain associated with sunburned skin, minor cuts, scrapes, insect bites and other skin irritations.
- **LavaDerm™ Cooling Mist** – may be used for cooling a fever or overheating.
- **Rose Ointment™** or **Animal Scents® Ointment** – pack in a small jar and use to sooth cuts and scrapes.
- **Sensation™** or **Genesis™ Hand & Body Lotion** – keeps skin hydrated.
- **Thieves® Cough Drops** - dry scratching sore throat or cough.
- **Thieves® Lozenges** – use to soothe sore throat and ease coughing.
- **Thieves® Hand Purifier** – use frequently to combat germs.
- **Thieves® Spray** or **Thieves® Wipes** – Use to disinfect tray table, armrests, headrests, knobs, handles, buttons, linens, pillows, remote controls, telephones, etc.; may be used to soothe a sore throat in adults and teens.

ADDITIONAL OILS FOR TRAVELING WITH CHILDREN

While many essential oils are suitable for adults and children, the list below includes oils from the KidScents™ and Seedlings™ line of products specifically formulated for babies and young children.

- **KidScents™ GeneYus™** – helps children make the transition to a different time zone and supports brain focus during travel and fun-overload
- **KidScents™ Owie™** – soothes cuts, scrapes, and other boo-boos
- **KidScents™ Sleepylze™** – calming and helps baby adjust to new schedule when traveling
- **KidScents™ SniffleEase™** – eases respiratory and/or ear discomfort, may help ease jet lag
- **KidScents™ TummyGize™** – relieves a variety of digestive discomforts in children
- **Seedlings™ Baby Oil** – use to dilute essential oils for baby for topical applications

OTHER ITEMS

- Band-Aids® – for minor scrapes or boo-boos.
- Roll of toilet paper – When traveling to a lesser-developed country, an extra roll might be very useful! My daughter has been the delight of those traveling with her as she stood outside a bathroom dispensing a few squares of precious paper to those waiting in line!
- Small flashlight with a fresh battery – just in case of a power outage at your destination
- Small pair of TSA-approved folding scissors – for projects and a myriad of other handy uses, including opening your vacuum-sealed bags.

It Fits

Carry-on Only

WEEKEND TRIP WITH A CARRY-ON ONLY

Pack the following in a quart-sized baggie:

- 5 mL oils: **DiGize™, Lemon, Palo Santo, Melrose™, Mountain Savory, Raven™, Endoflex™, Thieves®, Stress Away™, Deep Relief™ Roll-On**
- **NingXia Red®** packets – pack enough for at least one packet per person, per day.
- 2 oz. bottle YL Conditioner and/or Shampoo (Hint: Typically, you will only need one hair cleansing in a weekend. If you have been using YL hair products for a while, a long rinse of warm water followed by conditioner may be enough.)
- 2 oz. bottle **Sensation™ Hand & Body Lotion**
- Sample packets of other skin care items needed. (These can be purchased in Beauty School boxes.)

READY FOR TAKE-OFF

Your seatbelt is fastened, your seat back is upright, and the tray table is put away. If you opened the tray prior to takeoff, you remembered to use some **Thieves® Spray** or a **Thieves® Wipe** to sanitize it, didn't you? If you are concerned that spraying **Thieves®** will cause too much undue attention, then create your own sanitizing wipes before leaving home. Moisten a paper towel with **Thieves® Spray** or **Thieves® Household Cleaner**. Place this and an additional dry paper towel in a small baggie. Use to wipe your tray table, armrest, and headrest. Don't forget the bathroom knobs, seatbelts, inflight buttons, elevators, etc. If you are traveling with children and happen to be carrying **Seedlings™ Baby Wipes**, you could do the same with these. Sound too paranoid? You can also protect yourself by applying **Thieves® Hand Purifier** before and after touching items hundreds others have touched. Remember, germs can live on surfaces for many hours or even days.

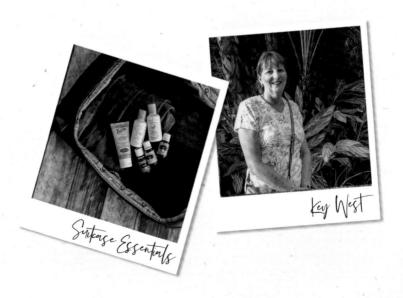

Suitcase Essentials

Key West

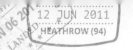

Symptom Guide

ATHLETE'S FOOT

Melrose™ essential oil contains two species of Melaleuca, alternifolia and naouli, along with rosemary and clove. This blend is especially effective for combatting fungi. If you are in a situation with communal showers, prevent athlete's foot by applying Melrose™ to the bottom of your feet as soon as you dry off. An inexpensive pair of flip-flops may also come in handy.

ALTITUDE SICKNESS

When traveling to mountainous regions, usually above 8,000 feet, you may experience altitude sickness. A lowered oxygen level is to blame for symptoms including headache, nausea, dizziness and muscle aches. When traveling to a destination of high elevation, altitude sickness may be prevented by avoiding activities that require physical exertion for a day or two after your arrival. Remain in your hotel and allow your body to adjust to the change before engaging in athletic excursions.

Peppermint and **Cedarwood** essential oils are both high in sesquiterpenes that help carry oxygen to the brain. Adding a few drops of **Peppermint Vitality**™ to drinking water may help alleviate symptoms. Cedarwood may be worn topically an inhaled often.

If you are prone to altitude sickness, consider taking O_2 drops found at local health food stores or online. These can be added to drinking water as soon as you leave for the destination and continually for the duration of your trip.

BEDBUGS

Contrary to popular belief, bedbugs are not a result of poor sanitation. They are hardy and good at hiding – they go where people go. Bedbugs are blood-sucking parasites similar to head lice, according to the Center for Disease Control, or CDC. They feed on human blood but are not known to spread disease. Bedbug bites are painless but can produce large, itchy welts.

Useful Prevention tips:

- In hotel rooms, use luggage racks rather than setting your bags on the bed or floor. Store luggage as far from the bed as possible.
- Hang all clothing. Leave nothing lying on the bed or furniture.
- Check the mattresses and headboards for signs of bed bug infestations before sleeping. Look for rust-colored or black stains along the edges of mattresses, especially between the mattress and headboard.
- If you find signs of bedbugs, check out and go elsewhere.
- Upon returning home, unpack your clothing directly into a washing machine, and inspect your luggage carefully. Vacuum suitcases thoroughly before storing.
- Spray interior of luggage with the Bedbug Spray and wipe the exterior of luggage with Thieves® Household Cleaner and spray it also.

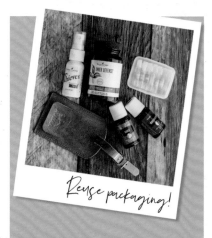

Reuse packaging!

HINT: MAKE SURE YOU LABEL ALL OF YOUR DIY CREATIONS PROPERLY. PLACE A PIECE OF CLEAR TAPE OVER THE LABEL TO PREVENT IT FROM BEING WORN OFF DURING YOUR TRIP. THERE IS NOTHING WORSE THAN CONFUSING A HOMEMADE THROAT SPRAY WITH YOUR BED BUG SPRAY!

TIP: I SAVE ALL OF MY EMPTY THIEVES® SPRAY BOTTLES. ONCE WASHED, THESE ARE PERFECT CONTAINERS FOR VARIOUS SPRAYS I PRE-MAKE, LABEL AND TAKE WITH ME ON TRAVELS. THESE CAN BE LEFT BEHIND TO MAKE ROOM FOR MORE GOODIES AND SOUVENIRS I FIND TO BRING HOME.

Bedbug Spray
10 drops **Palo Santo** essential oil
6 drops **Eucalyptus Blue** essential oil
5 drops **Cedarwood** essential oil
4 oz. distilled water

Combine ingredients in an amber-colored glass spray bottle. Use to spray bedding, carpet, upholstered furniture, linens, under mattresses, etc.

BLADDER/KIDNEY SUPPORT

When dealing with a kidney or bladder issue, it is important to drink plenty of fluids and avoid alcohol, soda and caffeinated beverages.

Combine 4 drops each of **Idaho Balsam Fir**, **Frankincense Vitality**™ and **Lemon Vitality**™ essential oils in a capsule. This trio is excellent for bladder and kidney issues, such as a UTI or even sudden pain from a kidney stone – that wants to pass on your vacation none-the-less. This combo may be taken as often as every 6-8 hours.

Ledum essential oil, also known as "Labrador tea" by Eastern Canadian people, has been used as a tonic for centuries to treat a variety of kidney-related concerns. Apply 2-4 drops topically over bladder/kidneys, or add to a capsule. Note: Ledum and Idaho Balsam Fir are not available as Vitality™ oils. Both of these essential oils have been consumed orally, even before the requirement of separate labels.

DIGESTIVE DISCOMFORTS
General Digestive Support

Peppermint Vitality™ essential oil alleviates all types of digestive discomfort, including overeating, heartburn, indigestion, bloating, etc. Place a drop on the tongue or add to water and sip.

DiGize™ – Rub over belly area for stomach discomfort resulting from food poisoning, diarrhea, gas or constipation.

DiGize™ Vitality™ – Take 2-4 drops orally, in drinking water or in a capsule, every 30 minutes until digestive complaint is relieved. One drop may be rubbed on the insides of cheeks or on tongue to stop a spell of dry heaves.

Overindulgence

JuvaFlex® essential oil blend, applied over the liver, can bring relief after you overindulge at the all-you-can-eat buffet or have a bit more alcohol than you should. Alternatively, apply one drop of **JuvaFlex® Vitality™** under the tongue or several drops in a capsule.

Ocotea essential oil promotes blood sugar balance, and is widely used as a digestive tonic. I routinely consume this oil orally when traveling even though it does not carry the Vitality™ label.

TACKLING MONTEZUMA'S MOUNTAIN

MONTEZUMA'S REVENGE IS A TERM USED TO DESCRIBE STOMACH SICKNESS RESULTING FROM DRINKING WATER THAT CONTAINS MICROBES WITH WHICH YOUR BODY IS NOT ACCUSTOMED TO DEALING. TYPICAL SYMPTOMS INCLUDE DIARRHEA, VOMITING, STOMACH CRAMPS, FEVER, MILD TO SEVERE DEHYDRATION, NAUSEA, AND LACK OF ENERGY. IF YOU ARE TRAVELING TO AN AREA WHERE WATER QUALITY IS QUESTIONABLE, IT IS WISE TO PACK A WATER BOTTLE WITH AN ATTACHED FILTER. USE THIS WATER FOR DRINKING AND BRUSHING TEETH, OR DRINK ONLY BOTTLED DISTILLED WATER IF AVAILABLE. IF YOU DO FIND YOURSELF STUCK HIGH ON THIS MOUNTAIN, HERE ARE A FEW TIPS: TAKE ONE INNER DEFENSE™ SOFTGEL EVERY 4-6 HOURS. TO REPLACE NUTRIENTS LOST THROUGH VOMITING OR DIARRHEA, SLOWLY SIP ON NINGXIA RED®. ALTERNATE BETWEEN USING DIGIZE™ ESSENTIAL OIL BLEND AND PEPPERMINT ESSENTIAL OIL AS DESCRIBED IN THE ABOVE SECTION.

NingXia + Inner Defense

Constipation – Keep things moving while traveling

ComforTone™ Capsules relieve travelers' constipation. Take one capsule with evening meal, increase daily until desired effect is achieved, then maintain as needed.

DiGize™ over the lower abdomen or **DiGize™ Vitality™** orally may also help get things moving.

Babies & Children

KidScents™ TummyGize™, applied to over the belly and bottoms of feet, will relieve a variety of digestive discomforts in children. **Ocotea** essential oil also aids digestion and is mild enough for children ages 5 and up, administered at one drop per quart of water.

EARS

Pressure changes

For ear popping or pain due to changes in cabin pressure, apply a drop of **Melrose™** essential oil blend behind the ear lobes. Chewing gum (**Slique™ Gum**) may also relieve pain and/or popping sensation. **Ledum** essential oil is another option that may relieve ear pain.

Babies & Children

Older children may use **Melrose™** for ear discomfort, but as it contains clove and rosemary, concerned mothers may substitute **Ledum**. A breast-fed child can be nursed during a flight, as swallowing will help combat ear popping. **KidScents™ SniffleEase™** may also bring relief when applied under the ears.

Earache

Melrose™, **Lavender**, or **Ledum** essential oil can help relieve ear pain from infection or swimmer's ear. Layer (apply one on top of the other) in this fashion: behind the ear, under the lobe and down the throat. And old-fashioned tip for swimmer's ear I learned from my parents is to place three drops of alcohol into the ear with the head tilted to the side. Count to ten and allow it to drain onto a tissue, and repeat with other ear. (Hint: plain vodka works for this and is readily available at bars. Purchase a shot and pour it into an empty 2-ounce bottle for use during your trip. Be sure to pack an empty bottle with dropper or at least an empty dropper.)

EMOTIONAL SUPPORT, INCLUDING FEAR OF FLYING

Soothing Stress, Calming Babies, and Promoting Restful Sleep

Lavender essential oil is a wonder for calming and relaxing both parents and children. Smell and wear as perfume to relieve stress while traveling. Add a drop to a pillowcase and a couple drops to the bottom of the feet to promote a restful night's sleep. Inhale or diffuse and wear on temples and across the forehead to relieve headaches.

To relieve anxiety, **Stress Away**™, **Peace & Calming**®, or **Tranquil**™ **Roll-On** may be inhaled, applied to pulse points, dropped on clothing or applied to the bottom of feet. All of these blends are gentle enough to wear around babies, and a drop can even be placed on the bottom of baby's feet. **White Angelica**™ essential oil blend also helps combat anxiety and over-stimulation. Inhale, diffuse, and/or apply to pulse points.

Frankincense essential oil can be inhaled to calm nerves, worn as a perfume, and used to anoint yourself and others during prayer.

Depending on your needs, **Valor**® essential oil blend can be either invigorating or calming. Inhale, diffuse, and/or wear on back of neck and/or bottom of feet.

Fear of Flying

Many people are afraid of flying. Others may not be afraid, yet it can still be stressful or frightening at times, especially when encountering extreme turbulence.

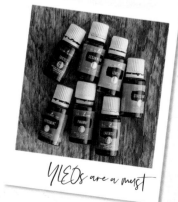

YLEOs are a must

But what if your job requires you to travel by plane? What if the family would love to go on vacation, and your fear of flying keeps you grounded?

I have personally been onboard two flights where I experienced issues severe enough for me to reconsider flying, but there are places I want to explore and my work necessitates some travel and rewards me with travel opportunities I do not want to miss. Flying often takes me to places I simply couldn't get to any other way.

Apply **Valor**® to pulse points, inhale deeply every 30 minutes of the flight. For added support, alternate with **Peace & Calming**® or **Tranquil**™ **Roll-On**.

Below are some suggestions of things you can do to make your flight less stressful and more delightful based on my own personal experience.

- If your fear is extreme, Google "getting over your fear of flying" for helpful ways to overcome your fear so you can enjoy our vast world of wonder.
- Pray before your flight and during takeoff. Thank God in advance for His protection and for giving you a safe and comfortable flight. Psalm 91 is one of my favorite Bible passages for dealing with fear.
- Carry and use the oils that are most calming to you, such as Stress Away™, Tranquil™, Peace & Calming®, or Lavender. Wear them and smell directly from the bottle during your flight. My personal favorite for this purpose is White Angelica™.
- Bring something to keep yourself busy and occupy your mind, such as watching a movie, reading a book, crocheting, knitting, or other portable craft or hobby. If I am not watching a movie as I crochet, I'll most likely be writing notes for my next project.
- Take a nap. If it's a long enough flight, take some relaxing oils in a capsule or SleepEssence™ softgels to help you sleep during the flight.

Babies & Children
Use **KidScents™ Sleepylze™** or **Lavender** essential oil to calm and help baby adjust to the new, temporary schedule brought on by traveling. Try adding a drop to the bottom of the child's feet or to the corner of bedding.

FATIGUE
Drink 2-4 oz. of **NingXia Red®** daily to combat travel fatigue and support the immune system. **NingXia Nitro™** provides a quick pick-me-up and promotes mental alertness without the sugar or caffeine overload of many energy drinks.

Apply **Valor®** to pulse points, inhale or diffuse to energize and invigorate. **Peppermint** essential oil can be also very energizing. Apply behind neck, or add a few drops of **Peppermint Vitality™** to drinking water.

FEVER & OVERHEATING
In the event of a fever or overheating, it is important to drink plenty of water. In some cases, medical attention may be necessary.

Peppermint essential oil can be applied to the bottom of feet and wrists to relieve a fever and cool the body. **LavaDerm™ Cooling Mist** may be used to gently mist the chest, arms, neck and face – with eyes closed – to cool the skin.

Babies & Children
For a feverish baby, place one drop **Peppermint** oil in navel, and cover with a shirt to avoid aroma overload.

FIRST AID
Boo-Boos, Cuts and Scrapes
Tsuga or **Helichrysum** essential oil will stop bleeding quickly. Apply liberally over the area, cover with gauze, and apply gentle pressure. Oils may be reapplied every 10 minutes if needed.

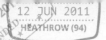
Assess to determine if stitches or medical attention is needed. Make sure to keep the wound clean by changing bandages daily.

For most cuts and scrapes it is a good idea to have a small jar of **Rose Ointment**™ or **Animal Scents**® **Ointment** handy. Alternatively, you may make your own blend. A good travel blend would include the oils of **Tea Tree**, **Tsuga**, **Lemon**, **Melrose**™, **Lavender**, and any others of your choosing (limit to eight essential oils total). Instructions for adding essential oils to Rose Ointment™ and recipes for homemade ointments are found in *The Art of Blending* (Debra Raybern, www.growinghealthyhomes.com).

Apply **Melrose**™ or **DiGize**™ to cuts and scrapes to disinfect before bandaging. **Mountain Savory** essential oil is another option that will prevent infection and speed healing.

Splinters

Thieves® essential oil blend can be used to draw out glass or splinters imbedded in the skin. Apply a liberal amount over affected area and bandage lightly. Reapply every hour until imbedded object is removable.

Tooth Abscess

For a tooth abscess when there is no dentist in sight, apply and ever-so-scant amount of **Thieves**® **Vitality**™ with your pinky finger directly to affected tooth. Note: Thieves® contains clove and cinnamon oils, which may be irritating to sensitive skin and tissue; dilute with a carrier oil if desired.

Babies & Children

Apply **KidScents**™ **Owie**™ to boo-boos. May top with **Rose Ointment**™ before bandaging.

HOSPITALIZATION*

It happens. We see it when we're at the airport: somebody returning home with a cast on an ankle, a brace on a knee or an arm in a sling. Having a few essential oils to help with minor and severe emergencies can help everyone cope with an unexpected event.

If you are unable to access the point of injury, you can still find relief from discomfort by applying oils as near to the location as possible, preferably the closest joint. Using oils you have on hand, such as **PanAway®**, **Lavender** or **Deep Relief™ Roll On**, apply every few hours for relief.

Refer to sections on First Aid, Emotional Support (stress), or other sections pertaining to your specific emergency.

IMMUNE SYSTEM SUPPORT
No Sick Days Allowed – Prevention is the Best Medicine
Protect yourself with **Inner Defense™** before and during your trip. Taken daily, this supplement protects the respiratory system against the flu, colds, and other communicable illness. Start taking one capsule daily a week prior to your planned trip. Continue taking 1-2 capsules daily while traveling. Inner Defense™ contains Eucalyptus Radiata essential oil, which helps maintain a healthy respiratory system when taken as a dietary supplement. After all, of the myriad of people you may encounter in confined spaces – plane cabins, train cars, cruise ships, or busses, not to mention where you will be lodging – someone is sure to have "the crud".

NingXia Red® supports healthy immune system function and combats a sudden onset of illness. Take one 2-oz. packet as needed, even as often as hourly for extreme issues. NingXia Red® provides a great way to squeeze in a little added nutrition while on your vacation or business trip. Rub 2-4 drops Thieves® essential oil blend on bottoms of feet before bedtime for an immune system boost.

After Inner Defense™ or Thieves®, **Mountain Savory** is my essential oil-of-choice to combat germs or unwanted pathogens. Take several drops in a capsule with water three times daily, or drop directly into mouth.

Babies & Children
Use **KidScents™ SniffleEase™** on the bottom of feet and/or on the back to relieve respiratory discomfort. Although it is already

diluted, you may combine with carrier oil, lotion, or **Seedlings™ Baby Oil** for further dilution on very small children or infants. **R.C.™** or **Raven™** may be used on older children; dilution will vary with each child.

INSECTS: IT'S A BIRD, NO IT'S A BUG!

Especially when traveling to another country, you may encounter bugs as big as birds! Well, maybe not *quite* as big as birds, but if you venture to areas of the jungle or rainforest, you are sure to encounter critters you've not seen the likes or size of before.

An excellent companion for keeping pesky critters away is **Young Living Insect Repellent**. While not permissible as a carry-on item, you can either transfer some to a smaller, approved container or pack it inside your checked luggage. I like to add several drops of **AnimalScents™ Infect Away™** to amp-up the repellent even more. You may also add 2-3 drops of **Purification®** essential oil blend to body lotion and apply to exposed neck, arms and legs.

Drink 2-4 oz. **NingXia Red®** daily to help alleviate allergic reactions to insect stings.

Bug Bite Treatment

Apply **Purification®** essential oil blend liberally to a bug bite. **Melrose™**, **Roman Chamomile** and **Lavender** may also be added to soothe the area. Re-apply every 15 minutes until itching and swelling have subsided.

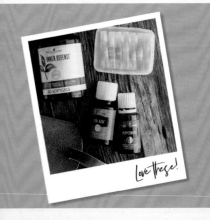

love these!

IF YOU ARE TRAVELING TO AN AREA WHERE THE TRAVEL BUREAU STRONGLY SUGGESTS INSECT AND MOSQUITO PROTECTION, REMEMBER TO TAKE A COLLARED, LONG-SLEEVED SHIRT, LONG PANTS, CLOSED-TOE SHOES AND LONG SOCKS. IT IS NOT WISE TO WEAR FLIP-FLOPS IN AREAS WITH SUCH WARNINGS.

Babies & Children
Kidscents™ Owie™ oil blend may be used alone or combined with any of the oils listed above.

JET LAG
Let's Take a Side Trip to the Island of Jet Lag
It's fairly easy to adjust to time zone changes of up to three or four hours. Simply stay up a little later and get up a little earlier without too much difficulty. When traveling a longer distance, subject to 9- to 10-hour time difference, I will go ahead and allow myself a cup of coffee to help me stay awake later and go to bed at a reasonable local time. Most often, re-adjusting once you return home is more difficult, and it takes a bit longer to return to a normal schedule. For some travelers, especially those traveling to areas with a vast time difference, jet lag can induce a variety of physical and emotional symptoms, such as anxiety, constipation, diarrhea, dizziness, coordination and memory loss or confusion, dehydration, headache, irritability, nausea, indigestion, and a general feeling of being unwell. Thankfully these symptoms are temporary, albeit annoying. Anytime you radically change your body's natural internal clock and sleep patterns, you may experience these symptoms. Giving yourself a full day of complete relaxation upon arrival will help your body adjust.

Lavender, **Peppermint** and **Cedarwood** essential oils are three good choices to help relieve jet lag. **Lavender** will promote sleep, even when you are not particularly sleepy. **Peppermint** provides a quick pick-me-up when exhaustion sets in and you feel you are ready to drop. **Cedarwood** will help with brain function. For each of these, inhale the oil and wear on the base of neck or scalp. To apply to the scalp, place a few drops in the palm of your hand, rub the fingertips of the opposite hand in the oil and massage into the scalp. The residue on fingers can be inhaled and rubbed onto the back of neck.

EndoFlex™ Vitality™ can also help relieve jet lag. Apply one drop under the tongue upon arriving at your destination.

NingXia Red® eases travel fatigue and symptoms of jet lag. Drink one 2-oz. packet as needed or hourly for extreme issues.

Babies & Children
KidScents™ **GeneYus**™ will help children make the transition to a different time zone and support brain focus during travel and fun-overload. Inhale, diffuse, and/or apply to the base of neck and temples. The oils in **KidScents**™ **SniffleEase**™ may also help when applied under the ears. **NingXia Red**® is for the whole family. As soon as they are able to drink from a cup, young children can enjoy a few sips of NingXia® in their water.

LYMPHATIC SYSTEM
The lymphatic system is largely responsible for removing the germs and pathogens the immune system has targeted for removal. When this system becomes clogged, it compromises the immune system and allows toxins to build up. The resulting buildup of toxins can lead to further infection and lengthen the time it takes the body to heal. Symptoms of a sluggish lymphatic system include: bloating, swelling, enlarged lymph nodes, brain fog, fatigue, digestive issues, and stiffness.

Apply one drop of **Ledum** essential oil under each ear lobe and down the throat to keep the lymphatic system functioning. May also be massaged along the spine or added to the Raindrop Technique® to drain congested lymph nodes.

Babies & Children
Ledum may be applied diluted to the bottom of the feet and/or spine of young children.

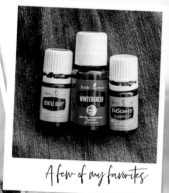

A few of my favorites

Ireland

MOTION SICKNESS

Dehydration can sometimes accentuate motion sickness. To combat motion sickness, be sure to stay well hydrated and smell **AromaEase**™ essential oil blend throughout the ride. Another option is to apply a drop of either **Peppermint** or **Ginger Vitality**™ essential oil to your tongue before departure and smell frequently during your trip.

MUSCLE PAIN: RECOVERING FROM FUN

Whether you have spent the day hiking, skiing, zip lining, or enjoying any other strenuous activity, at the end of the day your body can feel the effects of all that fun.

PanAway® essential oil blend soothes sore muscles as well as aches and pains. Massage a few drops over the sore area. **Deep Relief**™ **Roll-On** contains additional oils, including copaiba and vetiver, and is very soothing for aches, pains and joint stiffness.

Babies & Children

A parent can roll **Deep Relief**™ into the palm of hand several times, add a little lotion, and massage onto a child's back or other area where he indicates he pegged out the fun meter for the day.

PARASITES

Let's Take an Excursion to the Land of Parasites...

It's bad enough that you indulged on foods that upset your stomach and sent you "going" more times than usual, but now you picked up parasites and brought them home with you. Along with the stabbing, biting feeling in your abdomen, headaches, and indigestion, parasites can be serious business.

Worms and parasites can be found in the sand and soil, on animals, in food and in water. So what can you do to protect yourself from these invaders while traveling? This is another case where a little prevention goes a long way. After your trip, wash *everything* you took with you in order to prevent re-contamination. To sanitize shoes and other non-washable items, spray with **Thieves® Household Cleaner**, and if an item cannot be dried in a hot dryer, hang outside in the sun to dry.

During your trip and two weeks or longer after you return home, add two to six drops of **Ocotea** essential oil to your drinking water or NingXia Red® daily to guard against parasites. Ocotea has long been used for digestive concerns in South America and is great for protecting against and treating parasitic infections and as a digestive tonic. Less than one drop in one ounce of water daily for thirty days has been shown to eliminate parasites in young children.

Add one drop of **Lemon Vitality™** essential oil to drinking water daily to alkalize and purify. Many older essential oil texts list Lemon, taken orally, as a remedy to guard against malaria.

ParaFree™ is an adult formulation. Some adults, children, and those weighing less than 150 pounds will do better with Ocotea. (Note: ParaFree™ contains fennel. Some information states that individuals who are prone to seizures should not use fennel. Because Young Living oils are pure and unadulterated, this is typically not a concern. Many times our belief affects the way we react to a certain product or ingredient. However, if you still have concerns about the use of this supplement, consult your health care professional.)

IN CASE YOU GO...
FOR YOUNG LIVING MEMBERS WHO ARE FORTUNATE TO TRAVEL TO ECUADOR TO VISIT THE AMAZING GUAYAQUIL FARM, THE TRIP OFTEN INCLUDES AN OUTING TO THE LOCAL BEACH. IT IS BELIEVED THAT MANY MEMBERS HAVE PICKED UP PARASITES ON THIS EXCURSION. WEAR PROTECTIVE SHOES AND TAKE PRECAUTIONS TO AVOID UNWANTED PARASITES.

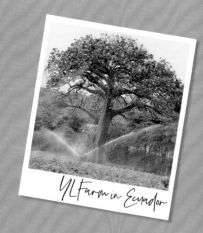

YL Farm in Ecuador

3 P's of Traveling Abroad: Parasite Protection Protocol

Parasite protection is especially important when traveling out of your country of residence or to areas where clean water is not readily available. You may increase the dosages below as needed, but if you use other precautions listed here, it is likely not necessary.

Beginning one-week prior to travel:

Begin taking one ParaFree™ softgel and two drops of Ocotea in drinking water daily.

During your trip:

Take one to three ParaFree™ softgels two times daily (2-6 softgels per day). Also increase to 2-4 drops of Ocotea daily. You may also add 1-2 drops Lemon Vitality™ to your water to purify. I take one ParaFree™ with breakfast and another with lunch. Six is a bit too much for me.

OH, I GUESS I SHOULD MENTION THAT SOME PARASITES GET REALLY ANGRY WHEN YOU TRY TO MAKE THEM LEAVE THEIR NEW HOME, A.K.A. YOUR BODY. THEY OFTEN RESORT TO BITING WHICH CAN FEEL LIKE YOU'RE BEING STABBED WITH SHARP DAGGERS. INCLUDING OCOTEA ESSENTIAL OIL IN YOUR PARASITE PROGRAM WILL HELP THEM TO LEAVE A BIT FASTER. IF YOU FORGOT YOUR OCOTEA, USE DIGIZE™ IN ITS PLACE. THE SECOND THING TO MENTION IS WHEN THEY LEAVE, YOU WILL OFTEN SEE THEM WHEN YOU USE THE BATHROOM. WAVE GOODBYE! BETTER OUT THAN IN, I SAY. A GOOD PARASITE CLEANSE MAY TAKE UP TO THREE MONTHS AS THE ADULTS CAN LAY EGGS ON THEIR WAY OUT.

Following your trip:

Following the instructions on the bottle, or adjust according to your need, continue taking three ParaFree™ softgels twice daily for a total of 21 days. Discontinue use for seven days and then repeat the cycle until the bottle is empty. Also continue taking two drops of Ocotea daily for 1-2 weeks after you return home.

Babies and Children

NingXia Red® is for the whole family. As soon as they are able to drink from a cup, young children can enjoy a few sips of NingXia Red® in their water. **Ocotea** essential oil is mild enough for children, administered at one drop per quart of water.

RADIATION EXPOSURE AKA FREE RADICAL DEFENSE

Passing through security x-ray devices is often a necessary security measure for travelers, especially in airports. These low-level electromagnetic scans may seem harmless, but any amount of radiation exposure carries risks. Radiation exposure may interfere with DNA replication and causes disruption of cellular communication, which in turn can disrupt the body's ability to protect and heal itself. The research varies wildly so I choose to be proactive and protect myself anyway.

Miso has a long history of research about its protective and restorative benefits after radiation exposure. When dining, ask for Miso soup. It's delicious and good for you.

NingXia Red® is the highest antioxidant liquid dietary supplement from whole food sources. Drink before and after exposure to radiation to combat free-radical damage. Several essential oils have been shown to possess antioxidants that combat free radical damage. Among those are clove, cinnamon bark, oregano, and rosemary. These are all found in the supplement **Inner Defense™**. Taking one capsule per day may provide protection not only from free radicals but also free-roaming pathogens, which can put a real damper on a vacation.

RESPIRATORY DISCOMFORT

Sore, Scratchy Throat

Palo Santo essential oil may be applied under the ears and on the neck to relieve a dry, scratchy throat. **Thieves® Lozenges** are very soothing and bring almost instant relief to a sore throat. In a pinch, if you do not have Thieves® Lozenges, you can spray a sore throat with **Thieves® Spray** for relief (teens or adults only).

Cough and Congestion

Grown and distilled on the YL farm in Ecuador, **Eucalyptus Blue** essential oil is high in eucalyptol, which is shown to be very calming to the respiratory system. It is the only variety of eucalyptus that does not cause allergic reactions in people with

allergies to eucalyptol. **R.C.**™ essential oil blend or **Thieves®
Cough Drops** may also be used to calm a cough.

Breathing Difficulty and/or Respiratory Infection
Apply **R.C.**™ or **Raven**™ to the chest and inhale or diffuse for
breathing difficulties related to high altitudes or at the onset of
respiratory infection. R.C.™ is widely used for respiratory support
and to relieve coughing. Though it may act as an expectorant
when applied to the chest, when inhaled via diffusing, it
promotes improved oxygen uptake and assists the body to
cough up mucus.

Babies & Children
R.C.™ or **Raven**™, diluted with a carrier oil or **Seedlings**™ **Baby
Oil,** can be applied to the child's back to relieve many respiratory
complaints. Alternatively, **KidScents**™ **SniffleEase**™ may be used.

SKIN
Keep Your Skin & Body Hydrated
When flying, pressurized air in the plane cabin can be very
drying. Other forms of public transportation, such as busses or
trains, may be full of stale air due to close quarters and compact
lavatories. This dry, stale air also wreaks havoc on your skin.
Always be sure to carry either **Sensation**™ **Hand & Body Lotion** or
Genesis™ **Hand & Body Lotion** in a small container for frequent
application. **The Bon Voyage Travel Pack** comes with many
travel-sized items. Carry a small container of your favorite Young
Living facial moisturizer to dab onto your face and avoid the dry,
shriveled look when you arrive at your destination.

Minor Skin Injuries
Apply **LavaDerm**™ **After-Sun Spray** to areas of sun-hot skin,
minor cuts, scrapes, insect bites and other minor skin irritations.
Apply liberally and repeatedly until skin is soothed and healed.

Babies & Children
LavaDerm™ **After-Sun Spray** may be used with babies and
children or can be substituted with **KidScents**™ **Owie**™.

The oils and products mentioned in this booklet only scratch the surface of the amazing line of products from Young Living™ designed to help us live at peak wellness all the time, even when on-the-go. Take the challenge to learn about one essential oil and one supplement every month. You'll be busy for several years learning about all of the possibilities the Young Living products give us.

Bon voyage!

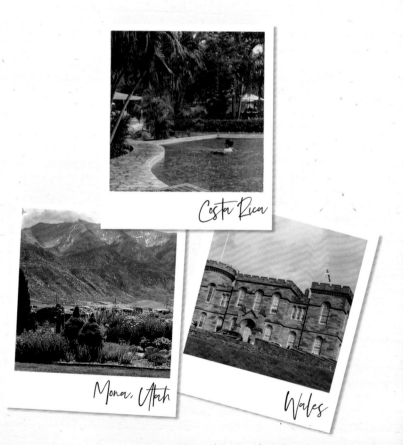

Costa Rica

Mona, Utah

Wales

Works Cited

Seppamaki, Kathryn. (2017, May 17). "18 Signs Your Lymphatic System is Clogged and How to Get it Moving Again!". *Functional Diagnostic Nutrition Certification Course*. Retrieved from: http://functionaldiagnosticnutrition.com/18-signs-your-lymphatic-system-is-clogged-and-how-to-get-it-moving-again/.

Transportation Security Administration. (Accessed on 2018, March 14). Retrieved from: https://www.tsa.gov/travel/security-screening/liquids-rule.

Watanabe, Hiromitsu. (2013, July 10). "Beneficial Biological Effects of Miso with Reference to Radiation Injury, Cancer and Hypertension". *Journal of Toxicology Pathology*. Retrieved from: https://www.ncbi.nlm.nih.gov/pmc/articles/PMC3695331/#r58

Essential Oils Desk Reference (EODR). Life Science Publishing. 2016.

Notes